PILATES
step-by-step

JUN 07

PILATES
step-by-step

How to strengthen and tone your body with fast and lasting results
·
300 step-by-step photographs and diagrams, plus special timed routines

Emily Kelly

southwater

This edition is published by Southwater

Southwater is an imprint of Anness Publishing Ltd
Hermes House, 88–89 Blackfriars Road, London SE1 8HA
tel. 020 7401 2077; fax 020 7633 9499
www.southwaterbooks.com; info@anness.com

© Anness Publishing Limited 2000, 2006

UK agent: The Manning Partnership Ltd,
6 The Old Dairy, Melcombe Road, Bath BA2 3LR;
tel. 01225 478444; fax 01225 478440;
sales@manning-partnership.co.uk

UK distributor: Grantham Book Services Ltd, Isaac Newton Way,
Alma Park Industrial Estate, Grantham, Lincs NG31 9SD;
tel. 01476 541080; fax 01476 541061;
orders@gbs.tbs-ltd.co.uk

North American agent/distributor: National Book Network,
4501 Forbes Boulevard, Suite 200, Lanham, MD 20706;
tel. 301 459 3366; fax 301 429 5746;
www.nbnbooks.com

Australian agent/distributor: Pan Macmillan Australia,
Level 18, St Martins Tower, 31 Market St, Sydney, NSW 2000;
tel. 1300 135 113; fax 1300 135 103; customer.service@macmillan.com.au

New Zealand agent/distributor: David Bateman Ltd,
30 Tarndale Grove, Off Bush Road, Albany, Auckland;
tel. (09) 415 7664; fax (09) 415 8892

A CIP catalogue is available from the British Library.

Publisher: Joanna Lorenz
Project Editor: Debra Mayhew
Designer: Lisa Tai
Photography: Christine Hanscomb (colour)
and Stephen Swain (black and white)
Production Controller: Don Campaniello
Editorial reader: Diane Ashmore
Illustrator: David Cook, Linden Artists

Previously published as *Pilates*

10 9 8 7 6 5 4 3 2 1

Contents

author's note

My aim in writing this book is to guide you through the Pilates technique in a stress-free and accessible way. I have always felt a huge passion for movement and exercise, and what I now hope to do is pass on some of that enthusiasm and energy to you.

When I started working as a fitness teacher, I tried to respond to my clients' individual needs by looking at all available types of activity and took courses in Alexander Technique, resistance training, swimming, circuit training, kick-boxing, boxercise, fitness assessment training, ante- and postnatal training, exercise to music, Indian champissage (head massage), self-defence, yoga and exercise counselling. I even tried line dancing!

△ **Regular Pilates practice helped me to correct muscular imbalances, made me stronger and leaner and reduced my risk of injury.**
Emily Kelly

I finally discovered Pilates after a visit from an American relative who had the perfect dancer's body: long and lean with fantastic elegance and posture. I endeavoured to find out everything I could about this technique so I took classes, studied and practised. To me, it was like "coming home": the moves were graceful and challenging and reminded me of the time I had spent doing ballet and gymnastics. I felt I was being taken back to basics and I loved the attention to alignment and the focus.

I became obsessed: every client had to try Pilates, and the results spoke for themselves. Everyone commented on the dramatic difference to their appearance, finding that their spine felt flexible and strong and their abdominals became flatter and tauter. Changes in posture brought about a more confident, slimmer appearance. What struck me as a teacher was how much people enjoyed Pilates, even the completely exercise-phobic. At whatever point you are starting, stick to this programme and your body will change, and this will have a balancing effect on your life. I wish you every success.

introducing
Pilates

In this first chapter we look at who can benefit from regular Pilates practice, why this book is different, and, most importantly, what you can expect to achieve. Refer to this chapter again when you feel that you need any additional motivation ...

If you have tried other exercise programmes in the past and wondered why their success has been limited, find out why Pilates is different and why its practice will become an essential, and enjoyable, part of your life.

introduction

Why another exercise book? What is it about Pilates that makes it such a favourite in gyms and dance schools and such a respected and popular activity? With all the different exercise videos and books on the market, what makes this book special?

Maybe the answer is in the book's title: commonsense. This book is designed to be an accessible manual that you can integrate into your life. It explains the key elements of Pilates and takes you by the hand through a comprehensive range of exercises. The programme aims to be very user-friendly: it is designed for beginners to Pilates but more advanced variations of many exercises are included so that you can set yourself a greater challenge as you progress.

The "first position" in each exercise is the most basic option. If you are new to Pilates then always start with this one, otherwise you will not have mastered the control and the focus needed to perform the exercise correctly. During a Pilates session your main concern should be the feeling that you get from doing the movement correctly, not how many repetitions you can do. The

△ **Pilates combines stretches and strengthening exercises, making it one of the safest and most effective forms of exercise.**

△ **Pilates help to re-define posture, creating a relaxed, confident stance. It is worth remembering that the correct posture can give an illusion of a 6 lb weight loss.**

"second position" should only be attemped after you have a clear understanding of the first position. For some people this may take two or more months. For others, it may take as little as three weeks. Everyone is different. It is not a competition, just progress at your own rate. The "third position" is a more intense variation still.

You may find that you progress faster with some exercises than with others. This is perfectly normal. For example, you may have a slight imbalance in your body that is being strongly challenged by the movement. Have faith in your knowledge of how your own body feels.

The holistic approach

This book aims to get you to look at exercise in a holistic way and to help you integrate it into your daily life with only minimal

disturbance. It does not set out to turn you into an Olympic athlete. It might, however, give you that little push you need to start exercising by explaining just why it is important, not just for aesthetic purposes but to help you avoid pain and injury, to make you feel good about your body and to increase your self-esteem.

The intention is that you will find the programme clear, logical and simple to remember, so that it will be quite easy to make it a regular part of your daily routine – just like brushing your teeth – because exercise really should be a matter of course. It's just common sense. You need to take care of your body at least as well as you take care of your car. You probably expect your car to last you six or seven years, and oil changes, tune-ups and wheel alignments are common practice for every car owner. How long do you want your body to last you?

Everyone can benefit

So who can benefit from this programme? Basically, Pilates has something to offer everyone, whatever your age or current fitness level. Although you will get stronger all over, one of the main benefits of Pilates is an increase in core strength. This is a phrase that is used over and over again in connection with Pilates, and it refers to the important abdominal and back muscles at your centre that support your whole body whether moving or at rest. As these muscles are strengthened, your posture will improve and you will find it easier to go about your daily tasks.

If you are completely new to Pilates, you will find these exercises different from others you may have tried. First of all, Pilates is a series of movements that flow into one another without pauses. Most conventional exercise starts and stops: you might do 12 repetitions of a move, rest, and then start up again with the next sequence. Pilates concentrates on the body as a whole, stretching some muscles, strengthening

◁ **Throughout the day try to give yourself a posture bodycheck. Try to pinpoint your bad habits as awareness is half the battle.**

more energy, extra alertness during waking hours and a general sense of well-being.

For the more experienced exerciser, Pilates can help to highlight imbalances throughout the body. The attention to detail and the concentration given to the movements can challenge even elite professional athletes, who often comment that they feel like beginners again after trying it. What appear to be the simplest of movements can be incredibly challenging when performed correctly, so do not worry if even the first position of an exercise seems hard to you: in terms of Pilates this is a good thing. As long as you work at your own pace, paying attention to how your body feels during the movement, Pilates is perfectly safe and very effective.

support and protect the lower back from injury, to help with general postural alignment and to allow the release of the hips for greater freedom of movement. Better core stability can therefore reduce the chance of injury. Improving it is often the way finally to get rid of niggling back problems that you may have suffered from for years. Core stability exercises are an important part of the Pilates method, which focuses on improving the strength and control of these stabilizing muscles.

The Pilates programme is very enjoyable and you should soon feel results which will motivate you to continue. If you adhere to it, you will be rewarded by improved posture, an enhanced feeling of balance, reduction in aches, pains and stiffness, greater flexibility and a longer, leaner, more highly toned body. As your posture improves, you will look as if you have lost weight, and one of the most frequently heard comments from people who are new to Pilates is that they feel "as if they have grown". This is because they have learned to lengthen up through the spine to its maximum potential, making them look slimmer and feel more confident.

Regular Pilates sessions will help your co-ordination and enhance your balance, which is of special importance through the

aging process. You will gain strength in a balanced way, so that tight, tense areas are stretched and weak ones strengthened. The realignment of your body will also make it easier for you to use it correctly. You will feel more relaxed and less stressed and will possibly benefit from other "by-products" such as more refreshing sleep,

▷ **Many osteopaths recommend Pilates to aid recovery and rehabilitation as well as a way of preventing possible imbalances or injuries. Remember though, if you feel pain or have an existing injury, always check with a medical professional before starting a new exercise programme.**

PILATES AND OSTEOPATHY

My introduction to Pilates followed a serious back injury. I was eager to recover as quickly as possible, and for the injury not to recur. I am a competitive runner (a former International 400m runner), so I did not want the injury to affect my training. I found a class and was impressed by the specificity of the exercises and how much more stable my back felt after several weeks of regular sessions. Since maintaining a regular regime, my back has felt better and my sports performance has improved. I now incorporate clinically based Pilates exercises into the rehabilitation of my patients and recommend it to them as an excellent way to improve their own stability.

Alex Fugallo
DO, ND, Bsc (Hons) Osteopathic Medicine
Registered Osteopath

The exercise environment

It is important to "set the stage" for your Pilates routine, creating a serene environment that will not divert you from the mind-body connection. So, before you begin, block out any distractions and ensure that your exercise session will not be interrupted. Here are a few tips for preparing your exercise environment:

• Find a comfortable, quiet area to work in, where you will have enough room to lie down without hitting your head on the coffee table.

• Turn off your phone, the television and any other machines that might disturb your routine.

• Aim to create gentle lighting, using natural daylight if possible or a soft lamp.

• Burning essential oils can help to create the right atmosphere: try lavender if you want a relaxing, calming session or orange to uplift or invigorate. Lemon is refreshing and is said to aid concentration: simply experiment to see what suits you.

• It is important to use a good exercise mat. Look for one that will protect your spine when you lie down; it should be firm but have enough padding so you can't feel the floor. Make sure it is non-slip and long enough for you to lie on when you are completely stretched out.

• Wear comfortable clothes; cotton is best. Avoid tight elastic bands, but do not wear very baggy clothes: you will feel stronger and sleeker in contoured clothes which allow you to move and stretch freely.

• Listen to soft, relaxing music with no harsh sounds. New age or classical music works well. Alternatively, a recording of natural sounds or crashing waves might be a good choice.

• Try not to have a heavy meal before starting exercise of any kind. Digesting the food while you are trying to work your muscles could cause cramps or indigestion. Allow at least two hours after a main meal before exercising. If you are hungry before you exercise eat a piece of fruit to tide you over.

▽ **Create a spacious and comfortable area for practising Pilates. Remove any distractions so that you will not be disturbed and wear comfortable, streamlined clothes so that you feel in tune with your body throughout.**

Locating the transverse abdominis

Sit or stand upright, inhale and pull your stomach towards your back, imagining that you are wearing very tight jeans and trying to pull your tummy away from the waistband. This is what you will be doing during all the Pilates exercises.

△ **1** Lie on your tummy with your head relaxed and supported on your folded hands or on a small cushion under your forehead. Keep your head in alignment with your back and the back of your neck long, without shortening the front. Try to keep your hip bones on the floor and relax your shoulders.

△ **2** Inhale, then as you exhale pull your navel towards your spine, trying to create an arch under your abdominals. You may not be able to lift very far up at first: this is not important as long as you understand the concept. Gently lift your shoulders back and draw your shoulder blades down your spine.

△ **If sliding your shoulder blades down your spine is a baffling request, practise this subtle movement by standing up with your arms by your sides. Keeping your back straight, push your fingertips towards the floor. Do not force your arms down or lock them into position. Try to keep the shoulder blades close to the back of the ribcage. This is very useful for limiting tension around the shoulders, which tends to make you pull your shoulders up to your ears.**

△ **Every movement should be controlled via your abdominals. Keep bringing your attention and focus back to pulling your navel towards your spine.**

Neutral spine

A healthy spine has natural curves that should be preserved and respected but not exaggerated. The term "neutral spine" refers to the natural alignment of the spine. If you have any serious pain in your back, check with a physician before embarking on any exercise programme. The main curves are:

1 **The cervical spine:** the area behind the head, along the back of the neck, is concave; it should curve gently inwards.

2 **The thoracic vertebrae:** the largest area of the back curves very slightly outwards.

3 **The lumbar spine:** the lower back should curve slightly inwards; it should not be flat or over curved.

4 **The sacral spine:** the sacral curve is at the bottom of your spine and curves gently outwards.

It is important to allow the spine to rest in its natural position to prevent stresses and imbalances. During Pilates movements you

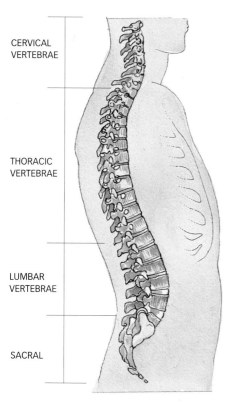

CERVICAL VERTEBRAE

THORACIC VERTEBRAE

LUMBAR VERTEBRAE

SACRAL

Finding neutral spine

The importance of neutral spine cannot be emphasized enough, as it allows your spine to elongate and relax. Before starting an exercise it can be helpful to roll gently between the two extreme positions and then try to fall comfortably between the two.

◁ **1** Tilt your pelvis, flattening your back into the floor.

◁ **2** Tilt your pelvis in the opposite direction, creating an arch under your lower back. Make this movement slow and take care not to hold for too long or you may cause tension in your lower spine.

◁ **3** Find a position between these two extremes in which your back feels natural and comfortable: this is neutral spine. Unless otherwise stated, you should always work from this position during your Pilates routine.

should ensure (unless otherwise directed) that your back is not flat or pushed into the floor, although this can be tempting in order to achieve a flatter tummy. What you tend to do in this position is grip at the hip flexors (the muscles located at the top of the thighs) thus creating tension in a place that is commonly tight anyway. You must also try to avoid over curving your spine, as this pushes the abdominals forwards and tightens the muscles around the spine. "Neutral spine" lies in between these two extremes and echoes the natural and safe position that your spine prefers.

◁ **The diagram shows the four natural spinal curves. These curves help to cushion some of the shock from our daily activities – even walking creates some mild stress. One of the key elements of Pilates is the close attention given to the alignment of the spine during all movements.**

Exercises for mobility

During the aging process, our range of movements can decrease making everyday activities harder, increasing our risk of injuries. The following exercises guide you safely and effectively through a series of exercises that challenge mobility, so helping to keep the joints healthy and flexible. Some of the exercises also challenge your co-ordination, balance and strength.

Rolling down the spine

Now you are ready to start your Pilates session with some mobilizing exercises. This is a really effective movement for mobilizing the spine, and can be very refreshing if you have a stiff back. However, if you have problems with your spine take advice before doing it. If you find it difficult you can do it with bent knees or against the wall, and you can also keep your hands on your thighs. Keep the movement flowing and remember not to collapse into it: the abdominals should not sag. During a Pilates programme, you can use this as a transitional movement to transfer from a standing to a floor exercise, so that the feeling of flow is not lost.

△ **1** Stand with your feet hip-width apart, balancing your weight evenly through your feet. Breathe in to begin and, as you exhale, lower your chin to your chest, and start to roll down towards the floor.

◁ **2** As you bend over from the hips, create a C-shape with the spine, letting the arms hang towards the floor. Feel your head relax and your shoulders drop. Don't sway backwards or forwards as you roll down. Make the movement flowing and controlled.

◁ **3** Start to curl back up, tilting the pelvis and trying to mobilize each part of the spine, uncurling it bone by bone and creating as much length as possible between the vertebrae. Try not to lean backwards or forwards but keep your weight in alignment, with your feet flat on the floor. As you come up to standing feel the crown of your head float up to the ceiling.

Purpose: To mobilize the spine and improve balance
Target muscles: Designed to loosen/mobilize the spine
Repetitions: Repeat 6 times

Checkpoints
- Create space between each vertebra
- Bend your knees and keep your hands on your thighs if required
- Create a C-shaped spine

▷

One leg circles

Circling the legs mobilises the hip joints and also challenges core strength, as you aim to keep the hips still during movement of the lower body, your thighs get a workout too. Keep the abdominals hollowed throughout. Make sure your spine stays in neutral and your shoulder blades glide down your back. The ribs may move away from the hips in this position so keep gently reminding yourself to control them. Make the circles flow and keep the movement continuous: think of a ballet dancer's grace and poise.

FIRST POSITION

◁ Lie on your back with your knees bent and your arms by your sides. Keep your spine neutral, your head aligned and the supporting foot firmly on the floor, raise one bent leg. Ensure your hips are square and still. Then start to circle your knee. Make small circles initially then larger ones, using your abdominals for control. The breathing for this movement requires concentration: break each circle into semicircles, inhaling as your leg crosses your inner thigh and exhaling on the outer edge of the circle.

Purpose: To mobilize the hips and build core stability

Target muscles: Adductors, hip flexors and abdominals

Repetitions: Circle 5 times in each direction, then change legs and repeat

Checkpoints
- Keep the hips square: don't let them lift from the mat
- Keep the spine in neutral
- Make the circle as large as you can safely control

SECOND POSITION

◁ Straighten the moving leg, keeping the other foot firmly on the floor. Lengthen up through your toes and try to make your leg as long as possible. If your hips start to move, you are not controlling the movement and would be better off continuing to work with a bent leg. Try to increase the size of the circle as you get stronger.

Checkpoints
- Keep the abdominals hollowed throughout the movement
- Extend the circle as you grow stronger

THIRD POSITION

◁ Straighten the supporting leg and lengthen, as if you were trying to reach the end of the room. Continue to lengthen up through the circling leg. Make the circles only as large as you can control. This position is really tough, so do not try to progress to it until you feel you have complete control in the second position. Remember to work from a strong centre.

Checkpoints
- Guard against over-curving of the spine
- Lengthen through both legs

The shoulder bridge

A very popular exercise in almost every class, this is a good mobilizer with which to start your session and a wonderful way to ease a stiff back. After this exercise your spine should feel loose and supple and it will also work your abdominals and lower body. The aim is for each bone in your spine to lift off the mat in succession. You may find that, to begin with, your back lifts in two or three sections: try to create length between each vertebra. As you lower yourself, place each vertebra in turn on the mat, imagining a pearl necklace sinking on to a velvet cloth.

The hips should be perfectly level, and you should try to create as much distance between your hips and your shoulders as possible. Do not forget to tilt the pelvis as you begin the movement. To mobilize the spine fully be sure to return to neutral as you lower your back to the floor, just before you tilt the pelvis and start the next lift.

Purpose: To mobilize the spine and challenge the abdominals

Target muscles: Erector spinae, abdominals

Repetitions: Repeat 6 times

Checkpoints
- Keep the hips level
- Maintain the distance between the hips and the ribs
- Make the movement flow

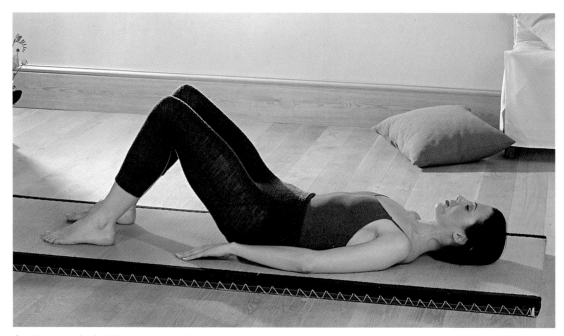

△ **1** Lie on your back with your arms by your sides, slide your shoulder blades down your spine and lengthen your arms away. Bend your knees and place your feet hip-width apart flat on the mat. Your head is in alignment and your spine in neutral.

▽ **2** Tilt your pelvis and lengthen the tailbone away. The whole length of your spine should be in contact with the mat.

△ **3** Slowly peel your spine up off the mat bone by bone, raising your hips towards the ceiling and keeping the abdominals flat and drawn down. In this position it is common to flare the ribs, so concentrate on keeping a constant distance between the hips and ribs. Make the movement smooth and flowing, inhaling as you lift and exhaling as you come down. Once you get used to the movement you can increase the stretch by taking your arms over your head.

abdominal and back exercises

The following exercises concentrate mainly on the abdominals and back – the staples of Pilates – although of course the body works as a unit throughout every movement. Feel the abdominals getting stronger, flatter and firmer as you progress and watch your wardrobe change. Your back will respond by allowing you to live your life in comfort and ease, free from the burden of aches and stiffness. Pay attention to the alignment of your body throughout the day, for optimum results.

Rolling back

Once you have mastered this movement, it is bound to bring back memories of childhood. We all rolled back and forth when younger and it did wonders for our backs. But do remember that it may not be as effortless now that your back has stiffened up – and make sure you work on a mat that gives plenty of support. Once you have practised rolling down the spine with your hands on the floor, try progressing on to rolling back: you may not roll back up on your first attempt, but keep practising. When pulling in the abdominals, imagine you are squeezing a sponge held between your navel and your spine. Squeeze the sponge as hard as you can. Take care not to roll back on to your neck.

Purpose: To mobilize and massage the back and strengthen the abdominals
Target muscles: Erector spinae, abdominals
Repetitions: Repeat 6 times

Checkpoints
- Keep your feet flat on the floor
- Lengthen up through the spine at the end of the movement
- Tilt the pelvis

FIRST POSITION

△ **1** Sit with your spine in neutral and your knees bent with both feet flat on the floor. Place your hands near your hips with your fingers facing your feet. Inhaling wide and full through the ribs, draw your navel towards your spine. Lower your chin towards your chest then, using your hands for support, start to roll down to the floor. Try to place each vertebra on the floor, one by one. To do this, tilt your pelvis and curve your spine into a C-shape.

△ **2** Once you have rolled down as far as you find comfortable, exhale and, using your core strength, return to the starting position. Pull up through the crown of your head to create a long spine, then repeat. Use your arms only as support and avoid transferring all your weight onto your triceps.

SECOND POSITION

Checkpoints
- Keep the chin tucked into the chest
- Do not grip the neck
- Use your abdominals to get you back to the starting position again

△ **1** Sit upright with your spine in neutral. Lengthen up through the spine and imagine your head floating up to the ceiling. Place your feet flat on the floor and your hands just below your knees. Don't overgrip: keep your elbows bent and your chest open. Take care not to tense or grip around your neck.

△ **2** Inhale as you tilt the pelvis and curve the spine into a C-shape to roll back, tucking in your chin and keeping your thighs close to your chest. As you exhale, use your abdominals to pull you back up to the starting position. Try not to use momentum, but make the movement flow at a consistent speed. Between each roll lengthen up through the spine.

SECOND POSITION

Checkpoints
- Do not tip the head forward or back
- Watch for tension in the neck

△ When the first position is understood, curl the upper body off the floor and continue the same movement. Let the chin fall towards the chest, and try to limit tension in the neck. Keep the hips very still, controlling any movement from the hips via your abdominals. Breathe laterally. Keep the stomach hollowed throughout the movement, trying to make it as flat as possible.

THIRD POSITION

Checkpoints
- Pull the shoulder blades down your spine close to the back of your ribs
- Lengthen the legs away
- The lower your straight leg, the harder your abdominals have to work

△ This position really challenges your co-ordination. As you raise the right leg, place the right hand on the ankle and the left hand on the inside of the knee. Change hands as you change legs. As one leg comes in to the body the other leg lifts and lengthens away on an exhalation. Keep your toes pointed and stretch down through the straight leg. The movement is controlled by the abdominals: keep them hollowed, and maintain the distance between the ribs and hips. Do not twist the hips: imagine they are being held in a vice. Keep the pace slow and consistent.

Leg pull prone

This is actually a yoga position as well as a modified Pilates position. You will gain a lot of torso strength and stability from this exercise, and if you do it properly it will feel as if every muscle in your body is being challenged. Remember to breathe freely throughout the exercise and do not hold your breath when holding the position. It is common to shrink down into your shoulders in this position so try to maintain the length in your neck throughout. Keep checking for tension around the neck, face and shoulders. Focus on your abdominals which should be stabilizing your whole body. You could try to visualize a drawing pin inserted through your navel and attaching to your back.

Purpose: To strengthen the abdominals and spine and challenge the upper body
Target muscles: Abdominals, stabilizing back muscles
Repetitions: Repeat up to 10 times

FIRST POSITION

◁ Lie on your front with your head in line with your spine. Bend your arms and keep your upper arms close to your body. Lift the abdominals off the floor, imagining that you are creating an arch under your stomach. Breathe wide and full. Concentrate on this abdominal lift and aim to hold it for one minute before relaxing again.

Checkpoints
• Slide your shoulders down your spine
• Keep the upper arms close to your body

SECOND POSITION

◁ Your elbows should be directly under your shoulders. Do not push your buttocks towards the ceiling or arch your spine. Keep your head in line with the spine and lengthen it away: don't sink into your shoulders or squeeze the shoulder blades together. Make sure that your hips stay square. The abdominals are lifted throughout. If this is too difficult, lower your hips and curl just your upper body off the floor. Try to hold this for one minute.

Checkpoints
• Maintain a straight line from your head to your knees
• Do not let the abdominals sag

THIRD POSITION

◁ Lift up on to your toes, straightening your legs. This is a real challenge, so be sure to have worked on the first and second positions for quite some time before progressing. Take care not to transfer all the weight into your shoulders or upper body, and keep your hips square. Pull your navel to your spine, maintaining the distance between your ribs and hips, and breathe laterally. Aim to hold for up to one minute.

Checkpoints:
• Keep a straight line from your head to your heels
• Do not transfer all your weight into your upper body
• Draw your shoulder blades down your spine

The side-kick

This is another good exercise for core strength, concentrating on the lower body. Have patience and work gradually through the progressions to achieve the best results.

When performing the Side-kick take care not to use momentum to lift and lower your leg. It may help to visualize moving your leg through mud as this will slow you down.

Your foot or knee should stay in line with your hip throughout the movement. Be aware of the alignment of your hips and keep them stacked on top of one another as it is common for the hips to roll forwards and the posture to collapse. This movement is stabilized by the abdominals and the obliques (the muscles at the side of the waist). Try to keep a constant connection with their involvement.

Purpose: To challenge core strength and work the lower body

Target muscles: Hamstrings, hip flexors, abdominals, stabilizing shoulder muscles, abductors

Repetitions: Repeat 10 times each side

Checkpoints
- Do not transfer all your weight into the arm in front
- Keep your abdominals flat

FIRST POSITION

△ **1** Lie on your side, resting your head on your outstretched lower arm. Keep your head in line with your spine, which is in neutral, and your hips stacked vertically: they must not roll in or out. Your knees are bent, one on top of the other. Place your free hand in front for balance but do not lean into the supporting arm or transfer your weight forward.

△ **2** Lift the top knee directly above the other knee. Inhale and, with your toes pointed, move the knee back as you exhale until it travels behind your body. The challenge is to keep your hips stacked and your abdominals hollowed. Your shoulder blades should be pulled down your spine and your ribs should not be pushed up. You should feel this in your side. If you want to increase the challenge straighten the top leg, keeping the toe pointed.

SECOND POSITION

Checkpoints
- Do not let the hips collapse
- Lengthen out through the legs

△ Straighten both legs. This is very challenging so be sure to advance only after working with the previous position first. Bring the bottom leg forward slightly from your hip, it should not be in line with your spine. Keep the hips vertical and lengthen out through both legs. The control comes from your centre. Exhale as the leg travels backwards.

The side-squeeze

This exercise will shape the waist and abdominals, so it is especially good for the area that hangs over your waistband when you wear fitted clothes. As you lift, check for tension in your neck or other parts of your body, and watch that your ribs stay down. Do not let the abdominals sag but hold them taut throughout.

If you wish to add an extra challenge, raise the top knee, keeping it in line with your hips – no higher. Make this a slow, controlled movement. Take care not to overgrip with your hands. Perform the movement with flow, avoiding any jerky movements when lifting and lowering.

Purpose: To strengthen the waist and mid-section, stabilizing and improving balance.
Target muscles: Obliques, shoulder stabilizers, abdominals and abductors
Repetitions: Repeat 10 times on each side

Checkpoints

• Do not allow the abdominals to sag
• Keep your hips stacked
• Maintain the distance between your ribs and hips
• Really feel the muscles in your side working

△ **1** Lie on your side with your knees bent and in line with your hips. Your hips are stacked and your abdominals hollowed. Place your hands on your head, directly opposite each other. Do not tip your head back or drop your chin to your chest. Breathe in.

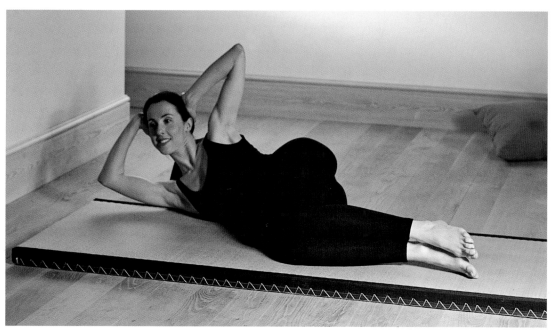

△ **2** Exhale as you lift your upper body off the floor and inhale as you lower. Make the lift slow and controlled. Don't jerk your neck or grip too hard with your hands. Maintain the length through your spine and take care not to let your hips collapse, but keep them stacked. Make sure your knees stay level with your hips. Draw your shoulder blades down your spine.

THIRD POSITION

△ **1** Drop your hips so that there is a straight line from your head to your knees. Your fingertips should be facing forwards and hands directly under the shoulders. Keep the abdominals strong and your hips square.

▷ **2** Exhale as you lower and inhale as you lift. Keep your head in line with your spine and forward of your hands. Don't let your ribs flare up. Keep your weight evenly distributed between your knees and your hands.

Checkpoints
- Keep a straight line from your head to your knees
- Do not let your buttocks stick up
- Do not arch or curve your back

FOURTH POSITION

Checkpoints
- Keep your shoulder blades down the spine
- Make it a controlled, flowing movement
- Breathe laterally

△ **1** Form a straight line from your head to your feet, supporting yourself on your toes and hands. The fingertips should face forwards and your head should be in alignment with your spine.

◁ **2** Lower your chest to the floor between your hands, then push up, keeping your elbows soft. Keep the movement controlled and continuous. Lower only as far as you can control.

Tricep push ups

A common complaint is the lack of muscle tone at the back of the upper arm: this is excellent for challenging this area. It works by adapting the classic push-up to work on the triceps. The movements may look the same but there are subtle – but very important – differences. The elbows stay close to the body this time. To help you keep your elbows into your sides, visualize doing the movement in a narrow space between two walls. Try to maintain a constant, and slow, speed throughout the exercise, although this can be very difficult to maintain on the last few repetitions.

Purpose: To strengthen the upper body and the abdominals

Target muscles: Triceps, pectorals, deltoids and abdominals

Repetitions: Repeat up to 10 times

Checkpoints

- Do not let your elbows "wing" out to the sides
- Watch for your shoulders moving up towards your ears
- Lengthen up through the top of your head

FIRST POSITION

▷ **1** Stand facing a wall. Place your hands flat against the wall, fingers pointing upwards. Your hands should be level with and just wider than your chest. Your feet stay flat on the floor. Keep your spine in neutral and slide your shoulder blades down.

▷ **2** Bend at the elbows to bring your chest towards the wall as you exhale. Unlike the classic push up your elbows should remain close to the body and pointing down at all times. Keep your head in line with your body and check that you are not pushing up your ribs. Push away from the wall to come back to your starting position.

SECOND POSITION

Checkpoints

- Keep your chest level with your hands
- Keep your head forward of your hands
- Keep your feet flat on the floor

△ **1** Position yourself on all fours, with your hands directly under your shoulders, fingertips facing forwards. Keep your spine in neutral and maintain a straight line from your head to your hips. Don't let the abdomen sag.

△ **2** Exhale as you lower your chest to the floor. This time, bend at the elbow and ensure that your elbows point towards your feet, with your upper arms staying close to your sides. As you push up, straighten the arms without locking the elbows.

One leg kick

This core exercise really challenges your co-ordination as you cannot see the movement – you just feel it. It is fantastic for toning up the lower body while challenging core strength. A good way to visualize the movement is to imagine that you are squeezing a pillow between your hamstrings and your calf. Try to resist just placing the leg: really feel the hamstrings working. This is a deceptively hard movement so do not worry if it takes practice. You may find it easier to get a feel for the movement first, then add the correct breathing pattern and work on lengthening down through the other leg.

Purpose: To tone lower body and develop core stability and strength

Target muscles: Hamstrings, erector spinae (when upper body is lifted), abdominals, gluteals

Repetitions: Repeat 10 times with each leg

FIRST POSITION

△ **1** Lie on your front, supporting your forehead on your folded hands to keep your head in alignment. Draw your navel to your spine, trying to form an arch under your abdominals.

△ **2** Relax the neck. Avoid clenching the jaw. Relax your shoulders and slide the shoulder blades down your spine. Bend one leg at the knee. This is your starting position.

Checkpoints

- Keep the movement swift and continuous
- `Limit any movement by keeping the abdominals hollowed throughout
- Slide the shoulder blades down your spine

△ **3** Inhale and, as you exhale, point your toes and make a stabbing movement with your foot towards your buttocks. Keep your knees together and lengthen through the legs.

△ **4** Ease out of this position then repeat, this time with your foot flexed. Then extend your leg back to its original position. Meanwhile, the supporting leg on the floor should be lengthening away at all times.

SECOND POSITION

◁ Perform the same movements, but this time curl your upper body off the floor and rest on your elbows. Slide the shoulder blades down. Keep your neck long throughout and watch that your ribs do not travel away from your hips. Lengthen through the spine. If you feel a pinch in your spine in this position, stay with the first position for a while.

Checkpoints

- Keep your neck in line throughout the exercise
- Breathe wide and full
- Do not push all your weight into your arms

stretches

Throughout your Pilates sessions you will be stretching and lengthening, but here is a whole chapter to take you by the hand through one of the most popular parts of most classes – the stretches. Notice how your range of movement will re-adjust, giving you more freedom and mobility in your daily tasks. Stretching is also linked to a reduced risk of injury – something everyone can appreciate. Many people notice a distinct "lift" in their mood after stretching, feeling refreshed and invigorated, with a general sense of well-being.

Spine stretch

If your back feels tight or if you just want a healthy and mobile spine then this is the stretch for you. You will feel longer, stretched and more flexible. This is a flowing movement, not a static stretch. To keep your spine lengthening up and to stop you collapsing into the stretch, imagine that you have a beach ball in front of you, and lift up and over the ball. As you come upright again, imagine that your back is rolling up a pole, vertebra by vertebra, and take care to keep this alignment from your head to your hips: do not lean forwards or away from the imaginary pole.

Purpose: To stretch the spine

Target muscles: Erector spinae, hamstrings, adductors and abdominals

Repetitions: Repeat 10 times

Checkpoints
- Do not collapse into the stretch
- Keep the movement flowing and continuous
- Let your head float up to the ceiling

FIRST POSITION

△ **1** Sit upright with your knees bent and your feet flat on the floor. Create as much length through your spine as possible. Keep the shoulders relaxed.

△ **2** Let your chin gently drop to your chest, then roll down bone by bone through your spine. As you do so, gently reach forwards with your hands. Keep your abdominals hollowed throughout. Roll back up to the starting position and lengthen up through your spine. Do not collapse into the stretch, but lift up through the abdominals and spine. Exhale as you lower into the stretch.

SECOND POSITION

◁ The movement is the same as before, but this time straighten the legs and flex your feet, lengthening the heels away. Bend the knees slightly if you find this uncomfortable. The legs should be parted as far as is comfortable. As you roll up create as much length as possible between the vertebrae. Keep your buttocks on the floor.

Checkpoints
- Do not have the legs too far apart
- Visualize reaching up and over a beach ball
- Roll up vertebra by vertebra

Spine twist

A deceptively challenging movement, this twist will stretch the waist and lower back while strengthening the abdominals. To gain the maximum benefit, it is important to keep your bottom on the floor throughout this movement. Let your head float up to the ceiling and pull your navel towards your spine. Try to keep the movement smooth and continuous. On your first attempts at this exercise you may be surprised how hard it is to sit correctly aligned. We all develop certain postural habits and this exercise challenges them so it will feel intense at first. It gets easier with practice.

Purpose: To stretch the sides, strengthen the abdominals and promote thoracic mobility
Target muscles: Obliques, abdominals, adductors and hamstrings
Repetitions: Repeat 10 times on each side

FIRST POSITION

△ **1** Sit upright, lengthening up through the spine, with your knees bent and feet flat on the floor, legs slightly apart. Cross your arms loosely across your chest. Maintain a straight line from your head to your bottom.

△ **2** Breathing laterally, inhale and, as you exhale, turn the upper body to one side, keeping your buttocks firmly on the floor. Repeat on the other side. Remember that this is a flowing movement, not a static position.

Checkpoints
- Keep the movement flowing
- Hollow the abdominals
- Lengthen up through the spine

SECOND POSITION

◁ The basic movement is the same but is performed with straight arms, lengthening out through the arms from the shoulders. Take care not to drop them. Now you are stretching in two directions: lengthening out through your arms and up through your spine. Slide your shoulder blades gently down your back and keep your feet flat on the floor.

Checkpoints
- Do not collapse into the movement
- Keep the whole of your buttocks on the floor
- Do not curve the spine

THIRD POSITION

◁ The movement is the same but this time straighten the legs and point your toes. You are now stretching in three directions: up through your spine, out through your arms and through your legs. Be sure to keep your buttocks on the floor. You may be tempted to lean into one side as you turn.

Checkpoints
- Lengthen all the way to the toes
- Feel the abdominals working

Lower back stretch

This is a good warm-up stretch. Taking deep breaths can help you to relax into the stretch and you may find your muscles becoming more pliable, allowing you to ease yourself further into the movement. The stretch is great for easing mild tension in the lower back, which is a common complaint. Some people find it beneficial to rock slightly from side to side while in this stretch as this can gently mobilize the lower back. To do this, keep your upper body on the floor and make the movement very subtle. Although a number of repetitions are recommended, these are only a guideline until you are confident about your instincts. Hold the stretch for longer or repeat if you need to.

Purpose: To stretch the lower back

Target muscles: Erector spinae and gluteals

Repetitions: Stretch twice; hold for 30 seconds each

Checkpoints

- Check for tension in the neck and shoulders
- Relax into the stretch
- Do not overgrip with your hands

FIRST POSITION

◁ Lie on your back and bring both knees up towards your chest. Support your legs with your hands, just below your knees. Relax your shoulders and feel the stretch in your lower back. Remember to keep your abdominals hollowed. Inhale to prepare and exhale as you lift your legs.

SECOND POSITION

◁ Curl your head and shoulders off the floor, imagining curling up like a ball. Keep your neck soft: do not force your head forwards to your knees. Take care not to overgrip – keep your elbows open.

Checkpoints

- Curl up and down slowly
- Make sure your mat is thick enough to protect your back

Spine press

This movement mobilizes and stretches the lower spine. It is a good one to try whenever your lower back feels stiff, especially if you have been sitting for a long period, at your desk for example (and it can be done very discreetly). The curve of the spine should be very subtle. Take care not to over curve your spine as you may "pinch" the muscles in the lower back. If it feels uncomfortable to curve your spine, or you have problems with your lower back, you may want to perform the second part of the movement only. When you tilt your pelvis, initiate the movement by imagining you are pressing your navel towards your spine. Avoid collapsing into the movement by lengthening your spine.

Purpose: To mobilize and stretch the lower back
Target muscles: Erector spinae and abdominals
Repetitions: Stretch twice; hold for 30 seconds each

Checkpoints

- Do not overcurve your spine
- Keep the abdominals hollowed
- Keep your head in alignment

△ **1** Stand a short distance away from the wall, with your back against the wall, your knees bent and your arms by your sides. Lengthen up and glide your shoulder blades down your spine.

△ **2** Inhale and, as you exhale, push your spine flat against the wall by tilting your pelvis and contracting your abdominals. Keep your head in alignment. Try not to collapse into the movement: keep your abdominals hollowed.

Simple stretches

The following stretches are great for lengthening fatigued, tense muscles. The two upper body stretches are great for opening up the chest; this is ideal if you have been sitting at a desk for a long period of time. On the first Chest Stretch, the wrist is also being slightly stretched. If this is uncomfortable, turn your hand round so that your fingertips point to the ceiling. In the Deep Chest and Back Stretch, slightly bend your knees if your legs are stretched beyond the comfort zone. When performing the gluteals stretch, be sure to keep your bottom on the floor or you will not stretch enough.

Chest stretch

This feel-good stretch is great for relieving tightness in the chest and uses the wall for support. It can be done almost anywhere to relieve tightness in the chest.

Purpose: To stretch the chest

Target muscles: Pectorals

Repetitions: Stretch twice; hold for 30 seconds each

Checkpoints
- Keep your spine in neutral
- Feel the stretch in your chest
- Relax your shoulders

△ **1** Stand sideways to a wall. Extend one arm and place your hand flat on it. Keep your hand in line with your chest and your feet in line with your hips. Draw in your abdominals; your spine stays in neutral.

△ **2** Now turn your hips away from the wall, so that you feel a stretch in your chest. Relax your shoulders and enjoy the stretch. Change sides and repeat the movement.

Gluteals stretch

This stretch is reasonably easy to do and promotes a greater range of movement in the lower body. It is also a valuable stretch to do before many different sports that involve a lot of lower body work.

△ **1** Sit on the floor and position one leg in front of the other (the legs are not crossed). Relax your arms in front of you. Lengthen up through the spine, creating space between the vertebrae. Don't worry if your knees don't fall to the floor, just relax and let the knees fall into a natural position.

△ **2** Drop your chin towards your chest and curl down the spine while pushing the arms forwards and keeping your buttocks on the floor. Curl up again, switch the positions of the legs and repeat on the other side. Do not collapse into the movement; keep the abdominals pulled in throughout.

Purpose: To stretch the lower body

Target muscles: Gluteals

Repetitions: Stretch twice; hold for 30 seconds each

Checkpoints
- Keep your buttocks on the floor
- Replace the spine bone by bone
- Create length between the vertebrae

Deep chest and back stretch

This stretch is ideal for easing tightness in the chest and back. Try to relax your shoulders and neck into the stretch. Remember, if this stretch is too intense, you can bend your knees.

△ **1** Stand facing the wall with your feet together and place your hands flat on the wall level with your shoulders, just wider than shoulder-width apart. Lengthen up through the spine.

△ **2** Inhale, then as you exhale lower your chest by bending from the hips, to feel a stretch in your chest and back. Keep your head in line with your spine. Keep the spine lengthened and the abdominals hollowed.

Purpose: To stretch the chest and shoulders

Target muscles: Pectorals and latissimus dorsi

Repetitions: Stretch twice; hold for 30 seconds each

Checkpoints
- Keep your head in line with your spine
- Keep your hips over your knees
- Bend the knees if necessary

▷

Abdominal stretch

This is a very popular stretch that is similar to the "cobra" in yoga. It is very good for stretching the abdominals after all the hard work they have done. Take care not to throw your head back in this stretch. Keep facing the floor and lengthen up through the top of your head to avoid sinking into the shoulders. If you feel any pinching in your lower back ease gently out of the stretch.

◁ **1** Drop your hips so that there is a straight line from your knees to your head. Glide your shoulder blades down your spine. Your fingertips should face forwards.

◁ **2** Inhale and, as you exhale, lift your upper body off the floor, resting the weight on your arms. Keep the abdominals hollowed and lifted, and take care not to overcurve the spine. Keep your hips on the floor. Do not sink into your neck, but lengthen up through your spine. Watch for tension in the neck. If you feel a pinch in your lower back ease out of the stretch.

Purpose: To stretch the abdominals

Target muscles: Abdominals

Repetitions: Stretch twice; hold for 30 seconds each

Checkpoints

• Do not overcurve your spine
• Keep your head in line with your spine
• Keep your hips on the floor

Hip flexor stretch

The hip flexors tend to be one of the tightest muscle groups, and when these muscles get overly tight they can cause discomfort and eventually imbalances. People involved in most sports benefit from this stretch, especially runners.

△ **1** Kneel down on the floor and take one step forwards, using your hands for support. If you need extra cushioning, place a pillow under the supporting knee.

△ **2** Lunge carefully into the front leg, exhaling as you lunge forwards. Make sure your raised knee is directly over your foot. Lengthen up through the spine and keep the abdominals hollowed. You should feel this stretch at the top of the rear leg. Change legs and repeat.

Purpose: To stretch the hip flexors

Target muscles: Hip flexors

Repetitions: Stretch twice; hold for 30 seconds each

Checkpoints

• Take care not to collapse into the stretch
• Lunge into the stretch
• Keep your head in alignment

Exercises to do during the day

Apart from your regular Pilates sessions, there are some exercises you can do quickly and easily wherever you are. Reassess your posture throughout the day and practise the key posture points: you could even pin up a list of these and check through it from time to time. Maintaining the correct posture in your Pilates sessions helps to re-balance the body and achieve optimum results.

Drawing in the abdominals

Whenever you get the chance, practise contracting your abdominals by drawing navel to spine. This action not only tones the abdominals but will get you used to the centring movement often used in Pilates exercises.

▷ Keep your back straight and in neutral. Inhale and, imagining that you are wearing a tight pair of trousers, as you exhale pull your navel away from the waistband, making your waist smaller. Lengthen up through the spine.

Wrist circles

If you have been working on a computer it is helpful to give your wrists a stretch to make them feel looser. Remember to take a short break from your typing or writing every 20-30 minutes.

◁ Start by circling your hand. Support it with the other hand at your wrist if this feels comfortable. Circle in both directions, making a slow, full circle. Remember to keep the spine lengthened and the abdominals strong at all times.

Hand stretches

If you are working at a computer, writing or doing any other kind of repetitive movement with your hands during the day it can be beneficial to stop regularly and stretch out your hands.

◁ Keeping your hand straight and somewhat taut, draw your fingertips down towards the inside of your arm. Use the other hand to press them gently down. Now turn your hand in the other direction, drawing your fingernails towards your forearm.

Drawing the shoulder blades down the spine

This technique should be familiar from all your Pilates exercises. Standing or sitting, bring your arms to your sides with the thumbs facing forwards. Slide your shoulder blades down your spine, keeping them close to the back of the ribcage so that they are not sticking out. If you are not sure if they are sticking out or not, you can deliberately do the opposite and make your shoulder blades stick out.

▷ By gliding your shoulder blades down your spine, you will reduce the effect of any tension you are feeling in your neck and shoulders. Although hunching your shoulders up to your ears is a common reaction, it will exacerbate any discomfort you are already feeling in that area. Try to maintain the distance between your ear and shoulder at all times, unless otherwise stated. Throughout the day you can monitor the tension in your shoulders and try to become aware of situations that make them hunch up. For example, it is common for tension to increase when working at a computer for long periods of time, or when using the telephone, but by becoming aware of your habits and posture you can make a conscious and effective effort at reducing tension.

Neck stretch

When we sit for extended periods of time, especially while typing or writing, it is common to experience tension in the neck and shoulders. If you do store tension in your shoulders, it can be helpful to shrug your shoulders up to your ears, hold ... then let go. The following neck exercises will help to gently stretch and mobilize the muscles around the neck to help ease tension.

△ **1** Keeping your spine in neutral and the abdominals strong, gently tip your head, letting your chin fall down towards your chest to feel a stretch in the back of your neck.

△ **2** Turn your head slowly from side to side, taking care not to overstretch. Keep your abdominals strong and your spine in neutral.

> ▷ Try to include lots of fruit in your diet. Carrying fruit around with you will mean you always have access to a healthy snack and are less likely to rely on high-fat, fast foods. Being organised, not obsessive, is a key factor in healthy eating.

(such as sugar and honey) metabolize quickly in the body and their energy is quickly "used up". The slower-metabolizing complex carbohydrates (such as pasta and rice) give you energy for longer periods of time, and at a much more even pace, maintaining a more constant blood sugar level than simple carbohydrates do.

Obviously, you should try to include more complex carbohydrates in your diet and fewer simple ones. The more refined (and usually sweet) a carbohydrate is, the simpler its composition. If possible, choose wholegrain cereals, brown rice and wholemeal pasta, which retain more of their original nutrients and also have the advantage of contributing fibre. Limit your intake of white flour, cakes and biscuits, as they tend to be high in sugar and fat. Also be aware that biscuits and cakes advertised as fat-free are not always healthier options as they can be loaded with artificial ingredients and sugar.

Fat is extremely concentrated in its energy power. One gram of fat equals nine calories; more than twice the amount of protein or carbohydrates. You need to take in fat for several reasons: it is an excellent, highly concentrated source of energy (a small amount of fat goes a long way, which was great for our ancestors but maybe not

such a prized quality today); vitamins A, D and E are stored in fat; it also makes food taste better and gives you a satisfied feeling. It is because fat tastes good that people end up eating too much of it and pumping many surplus calories into the body. Processed food manufacturers know this and add a lot of extra fat and sugar to their products to make them more appealing.

So how much fat should you consume? Most authorities agree that less than 30% of your total calories should come from fat. This may sound a lot, but almost all foods (including fruits and vegetables) contain some fat, so the calories keep piling up.

The average western diet contains around 40% fat. This, together with a lack of physical exercise, is the main reason for our spreading waistlines and the ever-increasing incidence of obesity-related illnesses. All foods will make you fat if you eat too much of them. However, fat will do the job fastest. The sum is simple: calories in (food) should equal calories out (activity). If one side of the equation does not balance the other, weight gain or weight loss occurs. All calories that are not used will be stored. However, the storage process is easier for fat

◁ Include as many vegetables as you can with each meal. There are so many different types now available that it is easy to experiment for variety.

calories than for protein or carbohydrate calories. Fat likes to end up on your body, waiting to be used on that unlikely day when there is no food to be had.

Fat is not intrinsically bad, but all fat is not created equal. Saturated fats contribute to the production of low-density lipoproteins, which cling on to the walls of your arteries, narrowing the passages and making them stiff and unpliable. The blood flows less freely and any particles that happen to be floating through can get trapped, possibly causing a heart attack or stroke. The message is to stay away from saturated fats. These are recognizable as they are almost always solid at room temperature, such as butter, lard and other animal fat. Some vegetarian products are also high in fat. Trans fats, found in margarine and some cooking oils, should be limited, as high consumption can lead to obesity and other debilitating illnesses.

Polyunsaturated fats are thought to help prevent skin complaints, heart disease and cancer. Essential fatty acids are present in fish oils, evening primrose oil, walnut oil and other polyunsaturates. Monounsaturated fats, found in olive oil, avocados, fish and nuts, are considered superior to other fats as they are linked to a decreased risk of heart disease, cancer and obesity. Most of your fat consumption should be from this last group.

Eating for life

Everyone has advice to give on eating, especially if it concerns losing weight, but very few can advise you on maintaining weight loss. Even if you find it easy to lose weight, it is very difficult to keep it off if you don't formulate a sound plan. Anyone can stick to a diet of grapefruit for a few days, or even a few weeks, but no one could or would want to maintain that kind of regime for the rest of their lives.

It can be psychologically traumatic for your weight to yo-yo. Not only must you cope with a sense of failure when you return to your average body weight, but those around you will perceive you as fighting a losing battle. It doesn't help you, but many take a great interest in other people's weight gains or losses.

When you lose weight rapidly through manipulating your diet - especially if your weight drops uncomfortably below your genetic size - and then inevitably return to your average body weight, the proportion of fat in your body may actually be higher than before. This is because some of the weight loss would normally have included lean muscle mass. Therefore you are making further problematic weight gain more likely, as lean muscle mass consumes more calories even when the body is at rest.

△ Try to involve your family and friends in your healthy eating habits. With their encouragement and support you are less likely to make poor choices. They may even have recipes or tips to share with you.

△ Create time to sit and eat in a relaxed manner. Eating in a hurry can lead to eating poor foods.

So what should you do if you want to lose some weight? First of all, you need to assess whether you really need to lose it. Not everyone is built like a supermodel: most bodies are designed with some extra padding, like a little warehouse ready for pregnancy or even for keeping warm in winter. No matter how hard you diet or exercise, you cannot fool your body's genetic programming. Those little fat storage areas are put there for a purpose; you may not be fond of them but they are part of your body.

This does not mean that you cannot improve your body. A sound diet and an exercise programme will make it strong. Your genes are a given but the way you treat your body will make a big difference.

maintaining your weight

The amount of calories you need to eat depends on how active you are. You want to keep fuelling your body; keep it happy and give it what it works best on. If you reduce your calorie intake too far, your body will interpret this as starvation and will react by slowing down its metabolism to save energy.

The main thing to keep in mind is that this is not a slimming diet - it is a way of eating for the rest of your life. It must be pleasurable and you must be able to lead a normal life. The plan is actually very simple: just avoid those foods that you know are high in fat and "empty calories" for most of the time and allow yourself a little more leeway for the occasional indulgence.

△ **There are so many excellent healthy-eating books on the market that it is easy to choose delicious but nutritious recipes.**

Reduce oils in your diet but do not avoid them completely. Extra virgin olive oil, for instance, is very beneficial, but fats, cheeses, and cream should be monitored. Alcohol (seven calories per gram) is another source of empty calories. This does not mean that you can never have another glass of wine: it just means that you should enjoy a glass of wine once a week instead of once a day.

Never say never again. That will only lead to frustration and anxiety. Chocolate is great, but it is very high in calories and should be enjoyed sparingly. Do not make it part of your daily diet but do not cut it out completely. If you do, you will end up dreaming about chocolate.

You should eat, and enjoy what you are eating. Food is one of the great pleasures of life. You should feel satisfied and not hungry or deprived. Think about filling up on foods that you can eat in larger quantities

UNDERSTANDING NUTRITIONAL INFORMATION

Try not to become obsessed with checking labels. Find products that taste good and satisfy your nutritional requirements, favour these then just check the labels of new foods. It can be psychologically damaging to over-analyse your diet – food should be enjoyed. Try to choose fresh, natural products, organically produced if possible. Beware of low fat processed foods as they can be full of additives, sugar and salt.

Fat

Food manufacturers may want you to believe that their products contain less fat than they really do. Take milk said to contain 2% fat. This actually means that fat makes up 2% of the total weight of the milk. But imagine a block of butter in a glass of water: if you measure fat as a fraction of weight, the butter (fat) is only a small percentage of the total. To measure the proportion of calories that come from fat, you need to know the total calories per serving and the weight of fat per serving. Take Brand X breakfast cereal:

Total calories per serving: 378

Grams of fat per serving: 14

There are 9 calories in a gram of fat, so 14 x 9 = 126. This is one-third of 378, so this product is 30% fat.

Calories

Calories are commonly listed in terms of serving size, which can be manipulated. The label on a chocolate bar may say it has 200 calories per portion, but there could be four portions in the bar. Some foods, such as avocados, are high in calories but also high in nutrients. Be sensible and base your choices on the percentage of fat, fibre and nutrients, rather than calories alone.

Sugar

Watch out for sugars that are not obvious, such as glucose, lactose or maltose. Of course, excessive sugar consumption not only causes dental problems but adds unwanted empty calories. A lot of fruit juices and carbonated drinks are full of sugar so try to stick to plain water for most of your daily liquid requirements.

Fibre

For a food to be classified as "high fibre" it should have a minimum of 5g of fibre per serving. Wholemeal foods, fruits, vegetables and pulses are all good sources. Fibre is important because it plays an important part in stabilizing weight and protecting against diseases such as bowel cancer.

without tipping the caloric equation. However, if you get the chocolate urge, go for it: anything else that you eat at that moment will not satisfy you. Just ask yourself if you really want to eat the whole bar or if a couple of squares would take away the

craving. Remember the 20% rule: if you only eat higher fat foods for 20% of the time you will feel less guilty. You will be surprised if you really start listening to your body. Most people in the west eat because of mental rather than physical hunger.

Make sure that you are adequately hydrated during the day: sometimes when you feel hungry you are actually thirsty. Aim to drink 2 litres/3½ pints of water a day (this can include herbal teas) as, among other things, this will give you the added bonus of healthy glowing skin. If you are going to indulge in a treat, try to eat something that has nutritional value such as nuts, rather than empty calories such as sweets.

◁ **Occasionally it is fine to eat foods that are high in fat. The key is balance. If you constantly deny yourself you will find your cravings increase.**

Frequently asked questions and answers

Will Pilates help me lose weight?

Losing weight – or rather fat – is a question of disrupting the energy balance, between calories in and calories out. A regular exercise programme will raise the body's metabolism, and although the amount of calories burnt per session may be quite small, over a period of time the average number of calories burnt will be greater. Pilates combined with a cardiovascular programme and a sensible diet will give you the results you desire.

I would like to get rid of the fat on my thighs and hips but every time I lose weight it goes from my face and breasts instead. What can I do to lose it from the right places?

Unfortunately, there is no such thing as spot-reducing. You cannot decide where you would like to remove fat, that is a decision that genetics takes for you. Many people think that by doing hundreds of abdominal exercises they will lose the fat around their middles but this is not the case. Just think about people who chew gum: if spot-reducing worked, they would have hollow cheeks! Instead of working incessantly on your lower body, you should also build up the upper body to draw attention away from the bottom half. Think what happens when you use shoulder pads - you look instantly slimmer.

I would like to start exercising again but last time I went to the gym I just got bulky and looked wider. I really dislike the current trend to be very muscular, can Pilates help?

Yes it can. Pilates builds long, lean muscles by keeping repetitions and resistance low. As it pays special attention to alignment, every move is designed to elongate as it strengthens, which is ideal for anyone who builds bulk easily. Think dancer's body rather than power-lifter's.

When will I start to see results? I have tried other programmes but I just cannot seem to stick with them long enough to see any real benefits.

If you are diligent about exercising and combine Pilates about three times a week with a cardiovascular programme and a sound diet, you should start seeing visible results within four weeks. Muscles you thought you did not have will peep through and your arms and legs will start to look more toned and streamlined. Your back will be stronger and your tummy may look flatter. However, the change won't only be visible. You will notice positive changes within yourself. You will start looking forward to your workouts and feel stronger in everything you do. You will sleep better and will most probably be in a better mood. Your aerobic sessions will become easier and you will be able to exercise for longer periods at a time. Give it a month: it's worth it.

△ Regular Pilates practice will improve your strength and flexibility.

I have quite a sway back (lordosis) and frequently experience back pain just above the kidneys. Will Pilates aggravate that situation?

Anyone with an injury or back problem should seek medical advice before starting this or any exercise programme. Pilates is an excellent technique for correcting certain postural deviations and strengthening weaknesses. However, it should not be used as a remedial method unless supervised by a trained and certified professional. Pilates will aggravate a situation such as the lordosis described above if the movements are improperly executed.

I am worried about incontinence (urine leakage) when I work out. Are there any exercises to prevent this?

The muscles of the pelvic floor can weaken, especially after giving birth. Like any other muscle, these can be strengthened to prevent the problem of incontinence. During urination, stop the flow a few times. The muscles you are using are the pelvic floor muscles and this action is exactly what you should do to strengthen them. You can do this anywhere: on a bus, at the supermarket, standing in a queue at the bank. Read the section on pelvic floor muscles for more information.

I play golf every weekend and find that I often suffer from a stiff back and neck after a game. Which exercises would be helpful in relieving or preventing this?

Pilates is an excellent training method for golfers as the customary action in this sport is quite often a hazardous one for the back. You should follow the whole programme, as all the movements will be beneficial. You may be pleasantly surprised as you discover that your game is improving with your improved strength and flexibility.

I have never exercised at all but would like to start with this programme. Could this be dangerous? I am a 54-year-old woman, slightly overweight and a non-smoker.

You should seek medical advice before starting this or any other exercise programme if you have any injuries or risk factors. These would include coronary heart disease, diabetes, high blood pressure, high cholesterol, obesity, a heavy smoking habit or a very sedentary lifestyle. Women over 50 and sedentary men over 40 should also check with their doctors.

I am extremely thin and would like to gain a little weight. What can I do? Won't Pilates just make me look even slimmer?

You probably do not get much sympathy from others as this is the opposite of most people's problem. Most bodies are genetically programmed to store fat, but yours is designed to stay very lean. Try to take in extra calories whenever you can, but do not rely on empty calories from junk food. Drink fruit juices instead of soft drinks and carry nuts and dried fruits or other high-calorie but nutritious snacks with you at all times. You should still exercise to build muscle, to give you a more toned, stronger look. Keep your cardiovascular exercise to a moderate intensity.

I cannot seem to motivate myself to exercise or change my diet. I'd like to lose some weight and get a more toned body but I lack the stimulus.

It is important to set goals that are realistic, measurable, and with a definite time frame. This will help you to look forward and stop you from seeing fitness as unattainable. You can set both long- and short-term goals. For example, "Within four weeks I want to be able to do the Hundred without having to stop halfway," is both attainable and realistic. Another motivational tool is to make a written agreement with someone who you know will support your exercise regime. Write out a contract stating that you commit yourself to exercising X times per week for X weeks. Have the other person sign as well as yourself.

◁ Although we are not suggesting that you walk around balancing a book on your head, we *are* saying that regular Pilates practice will improve both your alignment and your posture.

△ Pilates, combined with healthy eating and cardiovascular exercise, lengthens and stretches muscles creating a long, lean, strong physique.

Beware of people who may unconsciously want to sabotage your progress. Strange as it may seem, there are people who may not want you to succeed: friends who feel guilty about not taking care of themselves, mothers who are worried that you will do too much, jealous partners who worry that you will become too attractive to other people – odd, but true.

I am a single parent with no time for hobbies. I know I have to exercise but I often feel I have no free time.

When you have many demands on your time, it helps to examine all the reasons why you might choose to do something. Exercise can actually change your perspective, making you feel calmer and more in control. As they grow stronger, most people notice positive changes in their self-esteem and self-image. Headaches, backaches and depression can mysteriously disappear. With all these positive changes, exercise can become a treasured and necessary part of the day. Six weeks seems to be the point at which perspectives change. If you can reach a point where you feel you "want to" rather than "have to" exercise, it will take away the "chore" factor.

Don't forget that energy creates energy, and this will help you in your day-to-day activities. Pin up a big list of all the things that exercise will do for you, and keep it positive. For example, rather than saying "I want to be a size 10" say "I want to be confident and comfortable in my body". Do not underestimate the power of words and positive thought. Use affirmations to make you feel powerful. Sometimes it also helps to remind yourself that little is better than none at all, so start slowly and see what develops.

Glossary

Bone by bone

This term refers to the movement of the vertebrae, for example in the Shoulder Bridge. As a beginner, you may lift your hips from the floor in two or three stages. As you advance try to curl up the spine, working your way up each vertebra, lengthening and straightening as you go.

Breathe laterally

This is the best way to breathe in Pilates. Breathe wide and full into the ribs, taking them out to the sides as you inhale and bringing them back together as you exhale. Avoid breathing into the stomach or high into the chest as this can also involve lifting the shoulders and chest.

Core strength

This term is given to the muscles of the torso which control all core movements in Pilates. As these muscles get stronger and your core strength increases, your posture will improve.

Control

Only work within a range of movements that you can control. Do not use momentum to increase the range. This will not work your muscles to the same extent and may cause injury. Work within your capability and progress at your own rate.

Feet flexed

This is the opposite of pointing your toes. Pull your toes back towards the shin bone.

Flow

All Pilates movements should be smooth and continuous. To help maintain flow, imagine moving through soft mud. None of the movements should be jerky.

Glide the shoulder blades down the spine

During Pilates movements you should avoid hunching your shoulders. Practise by

first hunching your shoulders up to your ears and then slide them back down your spine until you create space between your ears and your shoulders and they are at right angles to your neck. This reduces tension at the neck and shoulders. Keep them here as you exercise.

Gripping

Gripping is the unnecessary overuse of the muscles, especially around the neck, hip flexors, feet, shoulders and lower back. This creates tension in the muscles.

Hips stacked

This term refers to the alignment of the hips when you are lying on your side, for example in the Side Kick. It is common to let the hips roll inwards or outwards. The hips should be balanced one on top of the other or you may create an imbalance.

Hollow out the abdominals

This is the basis of all Pilates movements. To hollow out your abdominals, imagine pulling your navel towards your spine, as if you were wearing tight trousers and want to create space between the waistband and your tummy by using the abdominals. Do not let the abdominals sag.

Keep the neck long

This term refers to the correct position for your neck as you exercise, as well as in daily life. Try not to shorten either the front or back of the neck by dropping your chin towards your chest or tilting your head backwards, unless otherwise stated.

Lengthening

This is the opposite of shortening your muscles, which may sound obvious, but it is something that most of us do all the time without realizing. For example, to lengthen your spine imagine a balloon positioned in the centre of your head. Picture it floating up to the ceiling and try to create as much space between each vertebra in your spine as possible.

Neutral spine

This is the term given to the spine in its natural state. To check if your spine is in the correct position, flatten your back to the floor then arch it. Neutral spine is the comfortable position between the two. This position protects your spine.

Ribs flaring up

This is something to avoid. The ribs should travel out to the sides as you breathe, *see* Breathing laterally. Maintain the distance between your hips and ribs rather than letting the ribs travel up towards the chest as this often involves arching the spine.

Tilt the pelvis

This term simply means pointing the pubic bone up towards your chin eliminating the natural lumbar arch.

Transferring weight

Take care not to distribute the weight of your body unevenly, for example in the Side Bend. You may be tempted to transfer your weight on to your upper body as this is easier. Instead, rely on core strength and use the whole body as a unit.

Useful addresses

Emily Kelly can be contacted at:

Synergy
Tel: 0208 200 6055

**The Global Independent Pilates
Reference Source**
PO Box 19344
London
W4 1GQ
UK

The Body Control Pilates Association
17 Queensberry Mews West
South Kensington
London
SW7 2DY
UK
Tel: 0870 169 0000 (office hours)

Balanced Body
7500 14th Avenue
Suite 23
Sacramento
CA 95820-3539
USA

Picture Acknowledgements
Superstock: 82R, 84TR, 84BL.

The Physicalmind Institute
1807 Second Street # 28
Santa Fe
New Mexico
87501
USA

**The Australian Pilates Method
Association**
PO Box 27
Mosman
NSW 2088
Australia

Body Studio
2/141 Wellesley Street West
Victoria Square
Auckland
New Zealand

Pilates websites are located at:
pilates.co.uk
www.bodycontrol.co.uk
www.michaelking.co.uk

GettyOne Stone: pages: 81, 82L, 83T, 83B,

Author's acknowledgements

Without the help of my associates and dear friends this book would never have been more than an idea. I would like to thank Michael King and Anoushka for being great teachers; Susan Newsom, Malcolm, Tiffany, Nikki, Saban, Jeanette Haslam, and Alex Fugello; and all my wonderful clients whom I consider to be close friends. Thank you to Tanya (for being so cool), Dawn (for making me happy), Debra Mayhew, Chris Mayoral, Louise Mulryan (for making me laugh), Nicola Jones (for her extraordinary tales), my sister, Heather, my loving parents, dearest Scott and, of course, my oldest friend and soul-sister Sharon. Thank God, for all my blessings and my treasured friends.

I would like to thank Valerie Foldvary who acted as an advisor in producing this book. The following is an outline of Valerie's qualifications and experience: Valerie Foldvary has been a respected member of the fitness industry for over fifteen years. She is a Reebok Master Trainer as well as an AFAA consultant. She holds certifications from ACE (American College of Exercise), AFAA (Aerobics and Fitness Association of America), ACSM (American College of Sports Medicine) for group exercise. She is a certified Personal Trainer and Lifestyle and Weight Management Counsellor and has also been a member of the educational committee for the revision of the ACE certification examinations for International markets.

Valerie, although of American nationality, lives in Madrid, Spain where she runs her own fitness consulting company, Californian Fitness Consultants. She writes fitness-related articles for several national magazines and has her own section on a weekly radio show dealing with health and fitness.

Valerie has been practising and teaching Pilates for several years. She conducts workshops for fitness professionals in both Spanish and English all over the world.

Index

index